Intentional Weight Management

Creating Radiant Health And Achieving Your Ideal Weight

Mahesh Subrahmanyam, M.Div.

Guha Services, Inc

Intentional Weight Management:
Creating Radiant Health and
Achieving Your Ideal Weight
By Mahesh Subrahmanyam, M.Div.

Copyright © 2004 Mahesh Subrahmanyam, M.Div.

Published March 2005

ISBN: 0-9768102-3-9

All rights reserved.

Reference to the Intentional Weight Management system, methods, and techniques is made herein pursuant to the express authorization of Mahesh Subrahmanyam, who reserves all rights. Materials fully describing the Intentional Weight Management system, methods, and techniques are available only through Mahesh Subrahmanyam subject to disclosure agreements.

Published by:

Guha Services Inc.

Cedar Rapids, Iowa

Phone: (319) 431-7131

Fax: (801) 409-3854

mahesh@guhaservices.com

www.intentionalweightmanagement.com

Printed in the United States of America

Table of Contents

Acknowledgments v
Introduction vii
1. The Big Picture 1
2. My Story 5
3. Super-Substance of Mind 9
4. Meditation 13
5. Using the Super-Substance of Mind 21
6. Putting It into Practice 27
7. Your Language—A Deeper Look 37
8. Subtle Language and Distinctions 43
9. Angelic Assistance 49
10. Why You Eat 57
11. Acid/Alkaline Bodies 65
12. Exercise 71
13. Observed But Not "Proven" 75
14. Diets Don't Work 81
15. Adding Weight, Also 85
16. The Final Chapter 89
Epilogue: Achieving Your Goals 95
Contract with Myself 99
Appendix: Acid/Alkaline Foods 101
About the Author 104

Acknowledgments

I love to acknowledge God, "Absolute Beingness," whose Grace is my conscious awareness and joy. It is God's Wisdom, Power, and Love that is contained in this book. If it were not also for all the assistance I have received from my Guardian Archangel, I would not be alive today to share this information with you. He has also helped me articulate this book on Intentional Weight Management for your benefit. He is my "soul friend" and it makes me very happy to be able to acknowledge him here.

My father and mother made many sacrifices to help get me where I am today. Their love and support throughout my life have been consistent and unending. My father's humor was also a great teaching—that love and humor continue to be nourishment that contributes to the blossoming of my present personality every day. I am very fortunate to have parents with hearts like theirs.

Without my wife, Yeelah, this book would have been impossible. It has been her belief in me as a writer, among other things, that has indeed supported the manifestation of this book. Her love and hard work allowed me to be at home and write this book for you. Her loving and caring heart expresses itself in her dedication to my joy and success. I love her beyond words; she is a priceless jewel!

Last but not least are all my friends who believe in me. They have contributed to my wisdom and maturity, constantly sharing their knowledge and feedback with me. They also contribute to the joy of my life in the playful ways they interact with me. My heart would be dry and less expressive without their involvement.

I am blessed in my life to have a relationship with all of the people and angelic beings I have mentioned; those in the spirit world and this one. These relationships have helped to develop my mind, heart, and soul. The grace I have received from all of them has added to the quality of my life in so many indescribable ways.

I trust that this book, which is a result of all that grace, will add to the quality of your life as well.

Divine Will Pleasure,
Mahesh Subrahmanyam, M.Div.

Introduction

Every day when I read articles or listen to the news, body-weight management appears to be a growing problem. In fact, it has been reported that obesity is reaching epidemic proportions. Many people are looking at this situation from various aspects, trying to find the reason and the solution. So far, however, body-weight management just seems to be getting worse, with no clear solution coming from those who claim to be authorities on the subject.

Many points of view exist for the source of the problem. Some say that a decrease in the levels of activity with an increase availability of food is the cause. Others say that a shift in the proportions of food types (proteins, carbohydrates, fats) we consume is the cause. Another group thinks food additives, from corn syrup to partially hydrogenated oils, are the cause. Finally, a small group of experts feels that more subtle additives, in the class of chemicals such as bovine growth hormone, are the culprits.

Different programs have been developed to address the possible causes. There are exercise programs that emphasize increasing activity levels while reducing caloric intake. There are diet programs that emphasize changing the proportions of the foods we eat. Yet other diet programs focus on removing all food additives and chemicals, and consuming instead only whole grains and natural foods.

Depending on your body type, most people get some short-term relief from one or another of these approaches. Others try combining different aspects from several diet programs and get some relief. But despite all of these various approaches, our weight problems still persist. Many people lose weight just to gain it back, plus additional pounds. Losing weight only to gain it back is the experience of the majority of our population.

So then what is the missing element that can address our increasing weight problem? What will allow us to manage our weight in a way that produces long-term results? How can we still have fun eating and have healthy, attractive bodies? What is the secret?

The secret is simple; "We are spiritual beings having a physical experience." We must handle our physical problems first on a spiritual level. This is where the real power for the solution to the problem can be found. This is precisely the level at which the system of Intentional Weight Management operates.

That is what this book on Intentional Weight Management is all about. In this book you will learn how to: (1) Achieve your ideal weight while having fun eating, (2) Increase your energy and alertness, (3) Produce a positive emotional state and, (4) Create a state of balanced health.

Remember, you never wait to manage your weight; you are doing it all the time, whether you know it or not!

Chapter 1

The Big Picture

Our physical bodies are a small part of a much bigger picture. We have a soul, a mind, emotions, and what oriental medicine refers to as a vital or energetic body. All of these aspects of ourselves are interdependent with our physical bodies.

We also exist within a much larger context. That context begins with our home and family. It also includes our friends and their homes. It extends further to our workplace, city, state, country, and world. It includes our thoughts, emotions, and environment, as well as the thoughts, emotions, and environment of our whole planet.

For thousands of years, ancient cultures have held the knowledge that everything is interconnected—"everything is related." Even Judaism, Christianity, and Islam tell us "God Is One," communicating to us our connectivity with a wholeness much larger than we can imagine. We have all experienced how our attitudes and behaviors affect our bodies, and how the attitudes and behaviors of others affect our bodies, as well. This is just a small glimpse into the larger context we all have with life.

Modern science is now finding the same thing that ancient cultures have known all along. Many articles appearing today, from environmental issues to physical illness and all the way down to quantum physics, report on the effect of life's inter-relatedness. In fact, some scientists report evidence that storms on the Sun affect Earth's weather patterns, satellite and cell phone communications, our moods, and even our behaviors, too.

So, even though we may imagine ourselves as separate, in reality we are connected within ourselves—physically, mentally, emotionally—and to the universe at large. Beyond that, we are part of something so majestic that no words can encompass it. This truth will be obvious if we just take the time to observe what is going on in our lives and the world around us. This observation can be disturbing and frightening as well as beautiful and majestic at the same time. When clearly seen non-judgmentally, this point of view usually inspires some form of action.

Narrowing the focus, our weight must also be seen in the context of our overall health. If our weight is out of balance, then other aspects that have already been mentioned, such as our mental and emotional states, must be out of balance, too. We cannot dedicate ourselves to achieve a particular weight no matter what the cost to our health. Anorexia, bulimia, and other eating disorders come from this kind of disturbing imbalance, dynamically impacting our overall health.

The approach we take to our bodies must be a balanced approach. It requires honoring our connectivity and maintaining the harmony among all aspects of our existence. It needs to provide the tools for producing good health, while at the same time allowing us to achieve our ideal weight. If we are going to continue to use this approach throughout our lives, it is necessary that it be joyful. These are the goals we focused on in developing the system of Intentional Weight Management.

Chapter 2

My Story

I grew up a chubby little boy even though I was very active. I went through emotional trauma, being teased by the children in my neighborhood. By the time I entered high school, I weighed 245 pounds and was very uncomfortable in most social settings. As fat people like to say, "It was all muscle." NOT! There was fat and plenty of it. I could not even bend over and touch my toes. I was extremely uncomfortable in my body and my mind. My emotions were totally blocked, and I was not in touch with how I felt most of the time. I did not fit in and life was very difficult.

Back then, I was not conscious of what was going on inside that caused me to be so fat. Now I have a clearer picture. Love for my overweight father caused me to model myself on him on all levels. This contributed to my being chubby as a child even though I was continually active. Also, some difficult sexual experiences when I was young made me extremely uncomfortable with the intense sexual drive I felt as a teenager. The experience of sexual energy was in direct conflict with what I believed was right for me to experience. The reason why I went to such extremes in my weight during high school was so I would not be attractive to the opposite sex and have to deal with situations that might arise, which in my mind were not okay. All the stress and the instability of my life—an overweight dad with heart disease, being uncomfortable with sexual energy, and later becoming involved with drugs—kept me overweight until my mid-thirties.

My overall health and weight began to change when I started to meditate regularly. The process of meditation began to address the underlying stresses and strains that put me out of balance. Slowly at first, and then more rapidly, I became conscious of my overall condition. I realized how uncomfortable I was in my body, mind, and heart. I also realized how my imbalances were preventing me from more enjoyable social interactions. With this realization, the door for change opened and I stepped through.

Not knowing how to work with my mind and body consciously, nevertheless, my weight began to normalize just from meditating regularly. At first it was a slow process. A clearer understanding began to emerge about sixteen years ago, and this made a big difference. As I worked more consciously to restore balance physically, mentally, and emotionally, my progress accelerated and I created a healthy body with an ideal weight. At the same time my, social dynamic changed and I began to enjoy life more.

Today my understanding has matured, and there is much greater clarity of the process I went through and how to share it with others. For sixteen years, I have maintained a healthy body with little effort. My weight now fluctuates between 145 and 150 pounds—quite a difference from the 245 I once weighed. One of my passions is gourmet cooking, and I eat chocolate almost every day. Still, my weight stays within a healthy range, fluctuating only about 4 pounds. Most of the time, I am emotionally balanced and have a reserve of energy from which to draw. I flow with the stresses of life in a more harmonious way, so they have virtually no side-effects on my health. In the last sixteen years, I have had three colds, the flu once, and no major illness.

The system of Intentional Weight Management was developed from the wisdom gained by going through my own transformation and by assisting others. In the following pages, you will learn how to work consciously to restore harmony and balance while creating a healthy body. This process will produce faster, long-lasting results that will normalize your weight. There will be many other benefits, such as increased energy, increased mental clarity, and greater emotional freedom that you will experience for yourself with this system. Let's move forward so you may benefit from the wisdom in the following pages.

Chapter 3

Super-Substance of Mind

I cannot say enough about how meditation helped me achieve balance and harmony, or how meditation has brought me to a place of greater conscious awareness. If it were not for my daily practice, I would not have the clarity of understanding I have today. Nor would I have recognized the distinction between myself and my thoughts and emotions. Meditation has increased my ability to discriminate between the real and the imaginary; it has helped put an end to judgment.

Beliefs give rise to attitudes, and attitudes give rise to behaviors. So when you see the illusion of your beliefs clearly, you can then replace them with beliefs that more accurately reflect reality. This process, in and of itself, helps to restore balance and harmony. It also produces attitudes and behaviors that are less likely to create stressful situations in your life. In fact, I have found that this process has produced much greater flexibility and has allowed me to experience life in a simpler more enjoyable way.

Your beliefs also create your physical reality in a very intimate way. It has been said by more than one source that the mind and body are deeply connected. It has also been said that everything comes down to "mind over matter." I like to say: "It is all mind over matter; if you don't mind it doesn't matter!" All kidding aside, the mind is a much more powerful tool than most people realize.

One thing needs to be made clear at this point—the mind is a tool we use to create. Whether you do it consciously or unconsciously you are always using your mind to create. It is not "you" and has no power over "you" … unless you allow it to be so. It was given to you to use for your benefit in creating a joyful life, a life of harmony, balance, peace, self-assurance, gratitude, and love. Unfortunately, most people, due to a lack of discrimination, are dominated by their minds and the thoughts and emotions it contains, rather than using the mind to their benefit. The people who have studied thought processes say you have millions of thoughts every day and most of them are repetitious and negative.

Medical science has discovered that thoughts create what are called neuropeptides. These chemical transmitters were first discovered in the brain but later were found to exist in every cell of the body. Quantum physics has also discovered that the mere act of observing something alters that thing in measurable ways. This is known as the "Uncertainty Principle." All this points to the fact that your mind is a very powerful, creative force and that the thoughts and the attention of your mind exert a powerful influence on your physical body and the reality you experience.

The missing links that most health practitioners and dietary authorities leave out of their corrective equations are:

- Deeply understanding the relationship between the mind and body
- Knowing how to consciously work with the mind.

If you don't adjust your beliefs and use your mind in a consciously creative way for change, then any small steps of progress you make will revert back over time. Your condition must return to its original state because the thoughts and attention that created the initial state of imbalance and ill health still exist. There is a direct chemical correspondence between your thoughts and the super-substance of mind that affects every cell in your physical body as well as the energy in your mental, emotional, and vital bodies. Unless you are interested in having three heart bypass surgeries, let's learn how to use our God-given resource.

Chapter 4

Meditation

I have already mentioned that meditation brought me to greater conscious awareness and increased my ability to discriminate between the real and the imaginary. I also mentioned how meditation helped me to realize that the mind is a tool for me to use and is under the dominion of my soul. Meditation also increased my ability to focus attention, as a laser focuses light. It is this kind of focus of attention, together with conscious awareness, discrimination, and several other factors that allows you to use the super-substance of mind most effectively. This being the case, the system of Intentional Weight Management starts with a meditation practice.

The simplest and most powerful form of meditation I have found is to meditate by gently placing your attention on your breath. Breath is the key to life, and mastery of life comes from mastery of breath. Dancers, runners, martial artists, painters, musicians, and even scientists who have mastered their fields, have mastered breathing while engaged in that activity. Ancient Hindu, Buddhist, and Taoist texts extol the value of mastering breath. Many physiological, psychological, and spiritual explanations are given for how your breathing affects your conscious awareness and your ability to function clearly in the world. Therefore, let's learn how to meditate using your breath and to enjoy the benefits.

It is good to prepare in advance to prevent your meditation from being disturbed. Find a quite place. Let the people around you know not to disturb you for the next 25 minutes. Turn off the ringer on your phone, turn off the TV, and stereo, too. "Silence Is Golden" so let your meditation time be your golden time. Give yourself permission to experience that "Peace That Passeth All Understanding." You do deserve this kind of oasis every day.

Next, sit in a comfortable position with your back as upright as possible. The idea here is to be comfortable and without straining. Maintain a posture conducive to mental clarity, not sleep. You don't want any sensations from your posture to take your conscious awareness away from the process of meditation itself. It does not matter if you sit on the floor or on a chair. It does not matter if you cross your legs or not. It is just about being comfortable yet alert at the same time.

Now that you are sitting comfortably and won't be disturbed, simply close your eyes and rest for about a minute or two. For now, don't even begin intentionally to place your attention anywhere; just rest and allow yourself to slow down. Sometimes it's helpful to take one or two deep breaths and let out a sigh of relief. This is your golden time now, a time for "R&R."

Now let's start meditating. Gently place your attention, your conscious awareness, on your breath. This is done simply, easily, and effortlessly, as when your attention goes to any thought that spontaneously arises in your mind. It is not a form of concentration into which you put effort. It is not a form of contemplation; you do not think about your breath. You just simply and innocently place your attention on your breath and allow your breathing to occur naturally.

During meditation, you are innocently and gently being with your breath, communing on all levels with its natural flow, surrendering to the process as it naturally unfolds, wherever it might take you. I like to start by saying, "Thy Will Be Done!" and then just let go and flow with the process. This is the most efficient attitude to have for this type of meditation.

Surrender and Trust are the keys. You are consciously surrendering the process to your spirit, guides, or what you perceive as God, trusting that the outcome will be to the highest benefit of all.

It is the experience of all people who practice meditation that their attention wanders during meditation. This wandering is natural and part of the meditative process. You do not try to control thoughts, you do not try to control your breath, and you do not try to control your attention by concentrating. It is even possible for your attention to be on your breath while thoughts are present. You simply have the innocent intention for your attention to be on your breath; and when you notice that your attention has wandered off your breath, you gently bring it back to the breath.

After you are finished meditating, relax again for about two minutes. Take one or two deep breaths during this time, and let out a sigh of gratitude. It has been your golden time, a time of "R&R," so appreciate the time well spent. Stretching out a little is good, too. I like to stretch my arms and legs out as far as I can. Then after about two minutes, slowly open your eyes. Now, you are ready to dive into activity refreshed and ready to go.

If you fall asleep during meditation, upon waking, meditate for about five minutes. When finished, follow the normal ending process for meditation given in the previous paragraph. This helps remove any grogginess that could persist from falling asleep during meditation. Meditation will release deep-rooted fatigue. Sometimes when this happens, we fall asleep. All practitioners have had this experience at one time or another.

You will probably be venturing into new territory with a regular meditation practice. You may want to stop meditating because at times it may become intense. There may be physical, mental, or emotional sensations that are uncomfortable. Such sensations are rarely dangerous, especially if you don't worry about them. If you find that the sensation is uncomfortable enough to distract your attention from gently being with your breath, then allowing your conscious awareness to be with the sensation for a time will quickly help release the stress associated with it. After the intensity dies down, gently bring your attention back to your breath.

Meditators have found it helpful to meditate regularly. This means twice a day every day, regularly for about twenty minutes plus starting and stopping time. If you meditate at about the same time of day, your physiology will get accustomed to traveling into deep states of restful alertness at those times. Most practitioners have found meditating before eating in the early morning and in the early evening the most productive times. Food can have too stimulating an effect to allow for deep meditation right after a meal. Meditating before sleep will often energize you so much that you will not be able to fall asleep for quite a while.

This is the simplest, easiest, and most effortless form of meditation I have practiced. It is a form that has been used for thousands of years by many different cultures. It is a form that can be done by anyone, almost anywhere, almost any time. It is a process that will broaden and add depth to your conscious awareness. It will increase your ability to discriminate and over time focus your attention the way a laser focuses light. It will cultivate your ability to use the mind as a tool to produce many benefits for your life.

Always remember to go easy with every step of the process, from setting up the preconditions, during the meditation process, and relaxing with the post conditions. Regularity and effortlessness are important and your success will be proportional to them. "Silence Is Golden" and you are naturally attracted to gold, so go for it. Just have the innocent intention and then let nature take its course. It's as easy as breathing and you naturally do that, don't you?

There are many forms of meditation that originate from many different traditions. Different types of people will be attracted to different types of meditation. If you already have a meditation process you enjoy, then please continue with your practice. You may want to try my suggested process of meditation, as well. What works best for any individual will depend on a variety of factors that are beyond the scope of this book to discuss.

One element I have found very important with all forms of meditation is your motivation. I experienced that meditating for gain and control do not produce successful results. One of my favorite statements that Buddha is reported to have said is, "I have gained absolutely nothing from Supreme Enlightenment, that is why it is Supreme." You already are Absolute Beingness, "Silent Singular Non-Localized Awareness" in Its total self-sufficiency. So there is nothing to gain and nothing needs to be gained. God the Supreme Absolute Being in its Total Wisdom, Total Power, and Total Love, is The Controller of all that exists. So meditating to gain control is an illusion of egotistic proportions.

The best motivation I have found is surrender to Absolute Beingness and Its Divine Will Pleasure. This attunes me to God's purposefulness for me. At the same time, it allows for me to dive deeply into my conscious oneness with the Supreme. This happens spontaneously by innocently and gently following the meditation process I have described. There are no moods, no contemplating, and no conscious effort to make anything happen or experience anything. It is simply a motivation that keeps me meditating, day in and day out, and has produced wonderful results beyond anything I ever imagined.

Chapter 5

Using the Super-Substance of Mind

I mentioned that meditation increases your ability to focus attention the way a laser focuses light. It is this kind of focus of attention, together with conscious awareness, discrimination, and several other factors, that allows us to use the super-substance of mind most effectively.

The three most important factors in using the super-substance of mind are: *attention*, *language*, and *imagination*. Conscious awareness and discrimination help you determine how and where to place your attention. To be fruitful, our attention must be simultaneously broad and focused. This is why regular meditation is so important.

In the beginning was the Word, and the Word was with God. God said, "Let There Be Light" and there was light. God, Absolute Beingness, is the ultimate conscious awareness and power of attention. His Word is the Supreme Language. His Imagination is The Light by which all things come into view. Now you can realize that you use the super-substance of mind to create, based on the same principles that Creation in its entirety is built on. The many different mystery schools that teach the fundamental principle that Creation is based on say: "As above, so below." You have been given the ability to use your mind in this same way. You just need to learn to cultivate the necessary qualities.

Just like God, the language you use is very important. You, like most people, probably have been unaware of how, moment-to-moment, the thoughts you have (your internal language) and the words you speak (your external language), shape your destiny. Your internal and external dialogues are so important because language shapes the quality of your attention. The shaped qualities of attention are what we call your imagination. This means that language is the cause of what comes into view for you. Your total language ultimately determines to a very large extent what you manifest and experience.

Imagination brings light to what it is you desire to create. "What you see is what you get," literally. The act of "bringing to light" is precisely what is necessary to create. Language is intimately connected to the quality of your imagination. Your choice of words, either internal or external, is exactly your choice of destiny.

Now that you know this, you must bring vigilance into the process. The vigilance I speaking of is to be continually consciously aware and discriminating about your total language. If you want to change, you must begin to examine whether the language you are using is, indeed, the way you really want to structure your attention and shape your destiny. For example, a woman who was going blind was unknowingly saying, several times a day, "I hate to see the world in this condition," or "I hate to see animal cruelty." By saying, "I hate to see," dozens of times a day, she was literally talking herself into blindness. And her subconscious mind was dutifully recording her every utterance as a blueprint for creating the reality she was experiencing.

You can understand the responsibility you have for your destiny. If you examine your life now in terms of your total language, "your internal and external dialogue," you will realize your responsibility in co-creating your life. This is a very freeing realization, because now you are empowered to author your life in a much more proactive way. You can now act from a place of conscious awareness, discrimination, and understanding. What is required is to locate the problematic language you have been using and determining the new beneficial language you want to substitute instead. Finally, be vigilant in substituting the new language every time you become consciously aware that you are about to use the old language. This will bring to light the results you desire in the same natural way that all of creation came to be. You have probably been creating your life so far in an unconscious manner. Now you really have an opportunity to be your own author of your life.

Many people who adopt this process realize that resistance does not work. If you try to resist your problematic language it just comes back more strongly. On the other hand, substitution works very well. When you notice problematic language (internal or external) beginning to occur, all you need to do is substitute the new language you have decided to use instead. It takes a little time to make the new language a habit. If you make the substitutions regularly, then the old language soon disappears and the new language becomes habitual. Resistance will only create friction, whereas substitution will create harmony and success. If you notice an error in your language has occurred, you may counter your mistake at that moment by substituting the new language immediately in your mind and/or aloud.

The implementation of this procedure may occur in stages that can be recognized with both internal and external dialogue:

1. Begin to discriminate about your total language.
2. You may notice yourself still using the old language spontaneously and only using the new language after the fact.
3. You may catch yourself in mid-thought or sentence using the old language and replace it on the fly with the new language.
4. You may notice the impulse to use the old language but before you start, you replace it with the new language.
5. The new language occurs spontaneously, having totally replaced the old language.

Let me assure you this process does require conscious awareness, discrimination, and vigilance. I guarantee that if you will make a commitment to working with the super-substance of mind in this way, you can transform just about any area of you life within reason. Let's see how you can use this process to transform your health and manage your weight.

Chapter 6

Putting It into Practice

In the course of my life, I have been fortunate enough to have met several master healers. One of them, Doc, is part of an ongoing network of researchers on the cutting edge of health. One day during a discussion about health and weight management, he mentioned that everyone has a set point for his or her weight. He told me that this set point was located in the hypothalamus, which is connected to the top of the pituitary gland in the center of the brain. He explained that many other types of set points reside in this area of the brain.

Doc suggested I do some research on my own, so the first place I looked was the available research. I discovered that the hypothalamus is a powerful part of your body's stability system. It strongly influences your emotional state, temperature regulation, hunger and thirst, glandular balance and function, sleep/wake cycles, involuntary nervous system, and many autonomous unconscious reactions. This was only the beginning. As I looked deeper into my own hypothalamus with conscious awareness and attention, I discovered to my amazement that, due to its being an anchor for the subconscious mind, many of my comfort zone set points such as prosperity, social closeness, and self-expression were also contained within this glandular region.

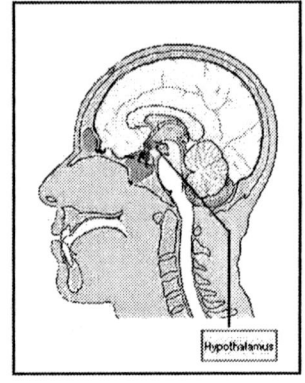

Armed with this information, I decided to put my conscious awareness into this area and change the set point for my weight. I sat down and meditated for a while, and then I entered directly into the hypothalamus with my conscious awareness. I intensely focused my attention on a particular weight of 160 pounds for myself. I internally languaged this weight, which gave rise to some images that I entertained in my mind's eye.

What happened over the next week was unanticipated. My life went into emotional and physical turmoil. All sorts of difficult emotions started to manifest. At times I felt very uncomfortable physically. My eating was unbalanced and not fun, either. I felt as if my life was spinning out of control. I wondered what I had done to myself and how I was going to get back into balance.

Having lived through many difficult experiences in my life has taught me to rely on an intelligence much more profound than my own. I decide to meditate and ask for help and guidance from God and my Guardian Archangel. What I was given next changed my life and the way I go about doing things. It altered the way I view my body and manage my weight. It improved my health and overall vitality. It brought greater harmony and balance to my entire life and revolutionized all my creative processes.

What was revealed first is that, for any activity to be totally life-supporting, it must honor your personal ecology. This means that all activity must match both the proper rhythm and proper force that your life follows. The rhythm and force are different for everyone and your own heart contains the knowledge of just the right rhythm and force for you. Whether you are working with the "super-substance of mind" to change some aspect of your life, or you are doing some kind of physical activity, choosing to push beyond your natural rhythm and force will be problematic.

The second thing revealed to me was that to try to manipulate your weight independent of your overall health is not life-supporting. Your weight is a function of your overall health. Sometimes what you think your weight should be is not the right weight for your overall health. I found this out the hard way. During meditation and prayer, I was given a clear way to enter into the hypothalamus, honoring these principles of rhythm and force. I was also given very specific language to use there to create a healthy body and spontaneously bring me to my ideal weight.

The process revealed was one of attunement to my heart. As I have said, through its natural beat, your heart contains the knowledge of the proper rhythm for your life. Your heart, through its natural blood pressure, contains the knowledge of the proper force for your life. Therefore, you must honor your heart and commune with it by becoming consciously aware of it. Then you can act in harmony and balance with your personal ecology and be successful. Every person's heart contains an enormous amount of knowledge. In fact, in some scientific circles, the heart is considered the second brain. I personally consider the heart to be my first brain, the seat of my intelligence, and the second brain up in my head to be my instrument for implementing the intelligence of my heart.

Before I describe the process I was given, I must share with you the language revealed so that you can attune to your heart and enter your hypothalamus to manage your health and weight. I was very surprised when it was given because I did not expect anything like this. Previous to being given the language, it was made clear to me that weight should not attempt to be controlled independent of health. So you can understand how powerful this simple language is: "RADIANT HEALTH." These two simple words are so powerful they have transformed my physical, mental, and emotional health simultaneously. They have managed my weight effortlessly. They have given me the freedom to honor the impulses that arise and to enjoy eating as I never did before. They have also led me to discover new things that have been very beneficial for my overall health.

If you look up the word *radiant* in the dictionary, you will find among other things: "beaming with brightness." If you look up the word *health*, you will find among other things: "soundness of mind and body." Imagine having a "sound mind and body beaming with brightness," this is *radiant health*. You would certainly be at your ideal weight under these conditions. This is the beauty of relying on a greater intelligence. I personally could not have come up with such a brilliant solution. (Pun intended!)

Now that you have the language you are going to use, let's go through what I call "The Radiant Health Process":

- Start by going through the premeditation process described in Chapter 4.

- Meditate for about five minutes or longer if you wish. I like to employ this process at the end of my meditation every day in the morning and evening.
- Gently place your attention on your heart, exactly like the instructions for meditating on your breath.
- After about a minute, have the intention to commune with the pace of its beat.
- When you have a sense of the proper rhythm for your life, then have the intention to commune with the pressure of its beat.
- When you have a sense of the proper force for your life, then begin to notice its gentle, yet powerful, influence in your whole system.
- Notice your heart's total connectedness to every part of your body—its fluid connection, the blood pressure, its rhythmic movement, even the sound of its beating as it moves through your whole body. (Realize the same total connectedness, force, and rhythm of your heart is a reflection of your entire life's preferred style, and is the wisdom and model for how you can best approach change in your health, body weight, and every other aspect, without exception.)
- Now gently turn your attention to the secret door at the back of your heart.

- Locate that door and place your conscious awareness in front of it.
- With the proper pressure/force for you, open that door.
- With the proper speed/rhythm for you, move through the doorway and follow the passage from your heart up to the center of the brain where the hypothalamus is located.
- In the center of your brain, gently place your attention on your hypothalamus.
- Bring your conscious awareness fully into your hypothalamus.
- Be still and observe what is going on here. What language is here? Who is speaking? Is the dialogue an accurate reflection of reality?
- After your observation seems complete for now, just commune with your hypothalamus for a few moments.
- Now, honoring your heart's wisdom, let the thought "Radiant Health" arise.
- Let this thought be in your hypothalamus harmoniously, "Thy Will Be Done."
- After 15 to 20 seconds, honoring the rhythm and force of your heart, again let the thought "Radiant Health" arise.
- Allow any images of a "sound mind and body beaming with brightness" to arise during this time also.

- Joyfully and lovingly embrace them with your conscious awareness.
- Continue doing this for however long your heart's wisdom dictates.
- When you're ready to leave, take a few moments to feel grateful towards your hypothalamus for accepting the new language/programming.
- Then gently leave and follow the passageway back to your heart.
- Take a few moments to express gratitude towards your heart for the wisdom you have received.
- End by going through the post meditation process described in Chapter 4.

Your heart knows just what is right for you. You may not feel comfortable completing the whole process the first time. I can't say what is right for you; you must be attentive to your own process and be willing to honor your own personal ecology. If it is right to complete the whole process, go for it. Most people find it very enjoyable and empowering, even the first time the process is followed. If at any point you have had enough, then follow the ending process for meditation. This is very important. Every step of the way, you must honor the wisdom of your heart to ensure safety and balance.

This process is very simple. At the same time, it is extremely powerful. It will have an enormous influence on your life. Overdoing this procedure can be dangerous to your health just like too much of any medication can damage your health. Any airplane is built to fly at a certain speed to reach its destination. If you attempt to fly it too fast, the wings break off and you never reach your destination. In this same way, you must honor the way you are built as you proceed on your road to change. Otherwise, you may never achieve your goals. I recommend you practice this process at least once per day, but please follow your heart's wisdom as to how often you do "The Radiant Health Process," especially at first.

Chapter 7

Your Language— A Deeper Look

Now that you have begun to observe your internal dialogue playing in the control center of your mind, you are capable of discriminating. An earlier chapter talked about a process for determining what language is incongruous with reality and replacing it with more suitable language. (Note: we do this outside of the hypothalamus process.)

As you live and breathe, on a daily basis millions of thoughts pass through your mind and you speak thousands of words in conversation. Here vigilance to "observe and replace" is very important also. Every thought and every conversation you have about your health and weight needs to be spoken in the same brilliant language if you expect long-term results. This is why it is equally important to be aware of and correct the language you use about your health and weight during the course of your daily activities. I also encourage you to continue to observe the interior language of your hypothalamus and continue working there.

Another revelation that came to me was the effect of thinking and speaking in terms of "losing weight" and my long-term success. This language has been powerfully problematic terminology for everyone. It ensures, for a majority of you, that your weight will return. Let me explain, so you can realize the importance of changing it.

Almost all of us from early childhood have been programmed to find what we lose. We have also been programmed to be winners, not losers. This is a society that rewards winners in a big way and puts down losers. Our slang phrase "YOU LOSER" indicates how much we want to avoid being a loser. Just look at any area in society—politics, academics, business, sports—everybody wants to be a winner. People are looking to gain in some way and keep what they gain. We all would like financial gains, economic gains, and social gain. (Some would like political gain.)

We have also been programmed to keep what we gain, to "hold on to it." Did you know that about 85 percent of the people who lose their car keys find them and about 85 percent of the people who lose weight gain it back—they "find it." How hard do you try to find whatever it is that you have lost? This is a part of your programming. So why on earth would you want to lose weight just so you could find it again and keep it?

If you are reading this book, you have probably gone through the process of losing and "finding" your weight several times. Please don't try to count how often, because you might get depressed. I know what it is like. I lost and gained many times—up and down like a yo-yo. Once I removed the concept of loss and gain from my internal and external dialog about my weight, then long-term success manifested. If you are going to have long-term success managing your weight, you must remove "losing weight," "lost weight," "I am going to lose weight," etc., from your language. You also must remove all language of "gaining weight," "gained weight," etc. These are very deep patterns in our society, and it will take vigilance to accomplish their removal. Everybody uses this type of language, and this is part of the reason there is such a large weight problem in our society.

Remember, the power of the word in the manifestation process cannot be underestimated. Your language shapes your attention and determines your destiny. For example, how many times do you hear a person say, "Every calorie I eat goes straight to my hips"?

The language I found that works best for me is:
- "Processing weight off my body and getting rid of it."
- "Processed weight off my body and got rid of it."

I have used this language both internally and externally for years. Even so, because it is such a pervasive part of mass consciousness, I slip occasionally. Still I remain vigilant and keep coming back to "Processed weight off my body and got rid of it" over and over and over again. This simple phrase has been like gold to me. It is priceless as far as long-term Intentional Weight Management goes. It seems so simple. It *is* simple, but it may take time, because you have been programming your subconscious mind with weight-gaining phrases for years. At the same time it works easily and most powerfully to allow the long-term management of weight.

I have shared with you the phrases I found that work best for me. Others have found that these phrases work very well for them, too. These may also be the phrases that work best for you. I am sure there are other ways to language around body weight that will promote long-term success. So please feel free to explore the language of your own heart. Your heart speaks its own language; all you need to do is listen. What you will hear will continually keep you in awe of the grand mystery of the Divine Intelligence that speaks through it. Peace, assurance, gratitude, and love are the responses people often have to its wisdom. Just remember your goal is "Radiant Health," so when communing with your heart, ask for language to support that!

Chapter 8

Subtle Language and Distinctions

Thousands of years ago, an Indian mystic and scholar named Patanjali did a lot of research into conscious awareness. He specifically focused on how language produced specific result. Pantanjali wrote an entire book on this subject that contains many formulas for producing some very interesting effects. These formulas are called "sutras" and are precise word combinations that are thought of silently in a quiet meditative state.

These formulas can be one word or a string of words. The formulas are not contemplated. Some of the results they produce are not obvious, based on the word or word combinations but, over several thousand years, these formulas have been verified to succeed. Many people have reported receiving the predicted results from these formulas, I being one of them. All you need to do is use the formula in the prescribed way and then the result comes quite naturally and spontaneously. These sutras are like seeds you plant with your focused attention and spontaneously fertilize them with your conscious awareness. Then they sprout and grow on their own within the natural cycles of time.

Patanjali reported one of these formulas specifically for controlling appetite and thirst. When used correctly, this formula regulates your desire for food. It will also spontaneously result in you eating the proper amount at mealtime. It allows for greater fulfillment of your hunger while eating the proper proportion of food. I have used this formula for years and can attest to its effectiveness.

The sutra for managing your appetite and thirst is: "Trachea." If you think about this word or try to figure out how it might affect your appetite, you are not going to get the results I have been talking about. In fact, your trachea is the tube that connects your mouth and nose to your lungs. It is in the front of your neck and only air goes into your trachea. Food and drinks go down a different tube called the esophagus, lying behind your trachea. From the point of view of pure anatomy, there would seem to be no connection between your appetite, thirst and the trachea. Nonetheless, this word, used in the prescribed manner, will affect you and support your overall health and Intentional Weight Management. The way to use the sutra "Trachea" is similar to the way we have already covered for using "Radiant Health" with just slight variation:

- Start by going through the premeditation process described in Chapter 4.
- Next, meditate for about five minutes.
- Then, gently let the thought "Trachea" arise in the same innocent way you think any other thought.
- After 15 to 20 seconds, again let the thought "Trachea" arise in the same way.
- Repeat this 20-second repetition for about 2 to 3 minutes.
- End by going through the post meditation process described in Chapter 4.

Remember, there is no concentration, contemplation, imagination, and no extra mental activity. Just innocently entertain the thought "Trachea" and then let it go. "Thy Will Be Done." That is all that is required of you for this process to work. Try it; it worked for me and may work for you. But keep it simple; any extra mental maneuvering will just inhibit the process and reduce the effectiveness.

This simple process done before meals will greatly assist in controlling your appetite. You can also use this sutra during the "Hypothalamus Procedure" after you have finished using the phrase "Radiant Health." Use it before meals for about six months and then just use it once or twice a day during your "Hypothalamus Procedure." This will work well to keep your appetite and thirst in harmony and balance with your radiant health.

You may recall that I discovered through research that the hypothalamus controls both thirst and hunger signals. I have noticed that some people have weight management problems because they eat when they are really thirsty. Distinguishing, through your conscious awareness, between the impulse to satisfy your thirst or hunger is very important.

One way to do this is to have the intention to make this distinction. Just knowing that your hypothalamus communicates both the impulse to drink and eat is the first step. Then, paying closer attention to the impulse is the next step. The next time you feel an impulse that causes you to start to grab some food, be still for a moment and ask yourself, "Am I really hunger or am I thirsty?" Many times you will discover that you are really thirsty. So grab yourself a nice big glass of clean water and in a short time you won't be hungry at all.

Drinking between six and eight 8oz. glasses a day is very important to Intentional Weight Management. It will keep you properly hydrated and prevent the opportunity of misreading the impulses from your hypothalamus. Water will also help you process weight off your body and get rid of it. It flushes out the waste materials from all your bodily processes. Drinking enough water is just good clean fun.

Remember, our bodies are a total of 70 percent water. Our brains are 80 percent water and our blood is 90 percent water. So consume enough good clean water to keep your system properly hydrated and you will see an immediate correlation in the quality of your overall health. You also won't eat when your body is really thirsty and your Intentional Weight Management will be that much easier.

Chapter 9

Angelic Assistance

If you use all the resources I have shared with you so far in this book, they will be of great assistance to you. Now I would like to share something that has been, continues to be, and will always be, that Supreme Resource. I am speaking of Divine Intervention. In many ways, Divine Intervention goes way beyond any other forms of assistance. I have experienced Divine Intervention as the resource that continuously leads me to all other resources. Let me share with you one of the ways Divine Intervention reveals Itself to me.

I want to tell you about your Guardian Archangel. That's right, *your* Guardian Archangel; each one of us has one. It is the Divine Will Pleasure of your Guardian Archangel to assist you on your life's journey. This specific Archangel has been with you from the moment God created your unique spark of conscious awareness—your soul. It has been with you in the realm of spirit every moment of your life. It has never abandoned you and is not capable of abandoning you anywhere or at anytime. Its purpose is to serve you now and in the future on your journey all the way back home to the world of spirit. If you believe in reincarnation, know that your Guardian Archangel has been with you through every life you have ever lived … and will be with you through all your lives to come. Your Guardian Archangel is your real soul brother or soul sister.

To receive assistance from this angelic being, all you need to do is ask. Its Divine Will Pleasure is in serving you. You must choose though, because in the Total Wisdom, Love, and Power of God, you have been given absolute self-sufficiency and free will. So your Guardian Archangel cannot and will not help unless you ask. Free will is a gift you have received from God, which your Guardian Archangel cannot violate. Cooperation is a choice you must make on your own.

A friend of mine shared with me today one of his mother's mottos, "The door to happiness opens outward." Indeed, once you open the door from the inside, unlimited joy may come into you. Without the door being open, it is very difficult for anything to get through. Those of you who have not opened this doorway are in for amazing grace and joy. After many years of living my life in this way I am still amazed at what continues to show up. The results I get in my life, the assistance that comes, the resources I am lead to, and most of what some might call "coincidence," come from the help of my Guardian Archangel and his Divine Friends. To me, a miracle is that which is being organized by powers greater than myself. Those powers, the Holy Agents of God whose orders are too numerous to count, are on your side and do want to help you on your life's journey.

You may be wondering, "When can I ask for help?" "How do I ask for help?" or, "What kind of help can I ask for and expect?" I have already answered the question, "Who do I ask for help from?" Your Guardian Archangel! I have answered the question, "Why do I ask for help?" Because you must ask, to be able to use this resource and receive an abundance of assistance that otherwise is unavailable to you. Ask because it is the Divine Will Pleasure of your Guardian Archangel to serve you, and to make your Guardian Archangel happy is your privilege.

So when can you ask for help? My Guardian Archangel sings this song for you now to communicate to you about "when" to ask:

Anytime!
When you get up or before you go to bed,
Anytime at all, you're always ahead.
Before you meditate and or after, too,
Just ask from a place deep within you.
Joy is in asking. Joy is in receiving.
Joy is in that which is beyond believing.
So whenever you ask, know that it's right,
Your Guardian Archangel has you in its sight.
Asking is no burden, it's what you can do,
In that fine moment, Divine Assistance comes through.
A twinkle in your eye, a smile on your face,
Grace has been given, to the whole human race.

There are many "right ways" for you to ask. Asking from a place of sincerity and trust works well. Coming from your heart with honesty and integrity is important. Using the specific designation of "Guardian Archangel' directs your request to the right place. You have to explore your own heart's joyful language that you can use in a focused consistent way. You can even ask your Guardian Archangel how best to ask. Believe me, you will be directed. Most likely there are as many ways to communicate with your Guardian Archangel as there are people and angels. I do know that making contact regularly builds a strong, clear working relationship with your Guardian Archangel. The more receptive you are to all possibilities of what may come through, the clearer and more complete the communication. Deeper realizations will occur when you come from a place of willingness to put your ego aside and follow the directions that are given. Asking with a sense of gratitude opens your heart and creates a state of receptivity. Allowing your Guardian Archangel to manage the details promotes a very deep level of surrender on your part. All of these are important clues and pointers to building your own unique relationship with your Guardian Archangel in the way that is most comfortable for you. Just start doing it and you will enjoy the benefits.

As with the "when" or "how" questions, I don't believe there are limits to the kind of help you can ask for or results you can expect. Obviously, by including this section in a book on Intentional Weight Management, I am revealing that I have used my Guardian Archangel to help with my radiant health and ideal weight. I have asked for specific diseases to be healed … and they were healed. I attribute much of my success with my radiant health and sustained ideal weight to my Guardian Archangel's assistance and guidance. In one form or another, the wisdom in this book has come from Divine Assistance, which is part of the reason I am presenting this material to you. There is nothing that you are limited to here. One of the ways my wife uses her relationship with her Guardian Archangel is to get a good parking place wherever she goes. As you may realize at this point, part of this whole process is in having fun, too. My

Guardian Archangel has a great sense of humor; you probably picked that up in the poem that came through. He once said to me, "Stay alert; life is a full contact sport." Lighten up; have fun; and don't be so serious. Be sincere, though, and you will get the results you are looking for.

I want to mention two things with which I continually ask for help, "Attunement with Divine Will Pleasure" and "Conscious Oneness with Absolute Beingness." When I surrender my will to God's Will, then I am the happiest because Divine Pleasure is part of God's Will. That is why I refer to it as Divine Will Pleasure. God's Joy for me is far greater than any joy I can create for myself out of my ego. It is my experience that Absolute Beingness is the supreme value of conscious awareness. Being "Consciously One" with that allows me to stay alert and play the game of life to the best of my ability. As you build your own relationship with Your Guardian Archangel, your heart will know what and when to ask for assistance.

Finally, I would like to mention that your Guardian Archangel is, in fact, a true Archangel. This is one of the highest orders of angels that God created. It is an enormously powerful being in "Attunement with Divine Will Pleasure" and in "Conscious Oneness with Absolute Beingness." It is God's Grace to give such a Soul Partner to assist you on your journey. This is a powerful presence that can accomplish many things, some of which are as yet beyond your imagination. Please keep an open heart and mind to this presence in your life, and ask for assistance. I guarantee you, it will be filled with grace and joy, keeping you in awe of GOD SUPREME.

Chapter 10

Why You Eat

As I mentioned earlier in this book, you are connected to your total environment. All the people you interact with—your family and friends, your workplace, city, state, and extending to include your world—are part of you. The collective consciousness of this world does have an effect on everyone in it, and everyone in it has an effect on world consciousness, which includes you.

You eat for a variety of reasons. Some of these reasons may be emotional. These emotions may be connected to the past or to the present. Part of being fat for me was dealing with the fall-out of past sexual experiences and the intensity of those feelings in the present. You, too, may be deeply motivated to maintain a certain amount of fat on your body to protect you from certain situations and the energy and emotions tied to them. For example, in one case, an overweight woman recalled in therapy that, as a seven-year-old girl, she'd overheard her grandfather say that the reason he'd survived starvation as a prisoner of war was that he'd been overweight, and his fat reserves had kept him alive while others had died. As a little girl, the woman had connected "fat" and 'survival,' thus programming her body.

You may have also developed some coping styles that involve eating food as a means of stuffing your emotions and not feeling. You encounter many people throughout the course of the day, and these encounters evoke many different emotions, some of which may be uncomfortable to experience for one reason or another. Eating, especially overeating, allows you to bypass these emotions for a while, instead of dealing with them as they arise. It is a way of denying what is real and living out your illusions. For many people, eating is a way of coping with stress. The world you live in today is filled with it. Family situations, work situations, and the state of the world all seem to be imbalanced and out of control. Stress is a huge component of your life and often food becomes a small but significant pleasure in the midst of many pains. It can temporarily stop the hurting. It may temporarily fill a void you feel from the apparent separateness of your life in today's world.

Other times, you might eat when you are happy or as a reward system. Done occasionally, this is not necessarily bad. However, if you find yourself eating too frequently or rewarding yourself for very minor things, you may be out of balance. This can result in short-term happiness that over time becomes a greater long-term sadness as you balloon into obesity.

Eating for emotional reasons never gives you what you are looking for. It really doesn't protect you. It really doesn't stop the feelings. It really doesn't fill any void. And it certainly doesn't give you any greater sense of connectedness to the ones you love or want to love. In fact, the result of overeating—becoming overweight or even obese—acts as a barrier to many of the things that would make you truly happy. For example, one woman, an avid traveler, was profoundly unhappy because her weight of 260 pounds limited her sight-seeing opportunities while she was traveling, so she spent $35,000 on weight-loss surgery.

This is why you must be vigilant enough to bring your conscious awareness to your eating. Whenever you have the impulse to eat, you can ask yourself, "What is the meaning of eating now?" If the answers were for any of the above emotions, then it would be best to allow yourself to feel the feeling rather than eating. It is a necessity to develop more coping skills than eating to deal with the situations that are uncomfortable and the emotions they stimulate. This will serve your radiant health because these emotions create neuropeptides that affect every cell in your body, whether you overeat or not. On the other hand, if the answer is, "my body needs nourishment," then give it the appropriate nourishment it requires.

What is the appropriate nourishment that your body requires? Most people have not really considered this question closely. The answer to this has supported my long-term Intentional Weight Management. There are two major categories for the nourishment of your physical, mental, and vital bodies. The first category is fats, carbohydrates, proteins, vitamins, and minerals that your body requires. I will speak more about fats, carbohydrates, and proteins in "The Final Chapter." The second category is the vital energetic component of what you eat.

Let me touch on the subject of vitamins and minerals for a moment. There is a wide range of opinions about vitamin and mineral supplements, and there are plenty of resources you can go to for your own research to help you decide what will work best for you. I will say, however, that over time, due to our commercial farming practices, our soil has fewer vitamins and minerals than it had thirty years ago. Therefore, foods that are being produced commercially today have a lot less vitamins and minerals in them. Your body requires a certain amount of each everyday, even more so now that life has become so intense and stressful. It stands to reason that your body hungers for these nutrients. By taking a moderate amount of vitamin and mineral supplements every day, along with smart food choices, my food cravings decrease and my long-term health is supported. I recommend a moderate nutritional supplement program to support your successful long-term health and ideal weight.

The second category of nourishment your body needs is the vital energetic component of what you eat—what the East calls chi or prana. You eat food for the vital energy force it contains. If the majority of the food you eat contains little or no vital energy force, then even though you might eat a lot of it, you will still remain hungry. I have observed how people who eat processed foods with little or no vital energy force continue to snack throughout the day. Their bodies are craving the vital energy force from the food that is being eaten. In search of this energy, they continue to take in more calories than their bodies require. This habit produces a fat, lethargic body. Have you ever wondered why some fat people seem tired even though they are putting plenty of "fuel in the tank?" Poor quality fuel produces poor quality performance in cars or people!

Some people believe that this force is contained at a very subtle level of the food. They believe that this level is the enzymatic level. The way food is cooked affects this level quite dynamically. Deep-frying food destroys most of the enzymes that a food contains as well, as its vital energy force. Any kind of deep-fried food contains little of the vital energy your body needs. Micro-waved food also contains little to none of the vital energy force your body needs. The intense internal friction that the food goes through during the microwave process destroys most, if not all, the enzymes and vital energy force your body requires.

The way many ancient cultures still cook and eat their foods today can be a good guideline to eating food with lots of vital energy force left intact. Stir-frying—cooking food fast on the surface without deeply penetrating the food with heat—maintains the food's enzymes and vital energy force. Cooking the food very slowly at low temperatures also maintains a large amount of the food's enzymes and vital energy force. Eating whole foods that are not processed and raw foods gives the body much more vital energy force. Uncooked, freshly sprouted foods have a tremendous amount of vital energy force. (My favorite is sprouted lentils, which I like to put in salads)

In my studies of Ayurvedic food science, I came upon information that the higher a food grows off the ground, the more vital energy force it contains. Maybe this is where the old wives' tale comes from, "An apple a day keeps the doctor away." A raw apple, which grows quite high off the ground, certainly contains a large portion of the vital energy force our bodies (physical, mental, and vital) require to sustain our daily activities. There are several successful alternative health clinics around the world and most of them use raw foods and juices as a big part of their protocol to energize the body.

I am not saying that you should never eat any particular type of food or eat only foods cook in a certain way. What I am saying is that you eat for total nutrition, and part of that nutrition is energetic. If you pay attention to eating for the vital energy force in food, then your eating remains in balance. If you don't, then you may find yourself hungry when you don't have to be. This can lead to consuming far more calories than your body requires. You may end up weighing much more than what is healthy. Do your best to pay attention to the vital energy force in the food you eat. This will help your appetite spontaneously finds its proper balance. Your energy will increase. You will have greater vitality and age more slowly. Now that is a really good thing, isn't it?

Chapter 11

Acid/Alkaline Bodies

The acid/alkaline balance of your body is a key indicator of your radiant health and ideal body weight. It has been discovered that the more acidic your body is, the less oxygen it contains. This causes you to feel run down and to eat more to try to acquire more energy. What your body really needs is to absorb more oxygen from the air you breathe, which happens when you are more alkaline. Over-acidity decreases the body's ability to absorb minerals and other nutrients, causing your body to break down in many ways, resulting in becoming disease-prone. This lack of absorption also results in deep food cravings.

The acid/alkaline factor is of primary importance to most of the world's ancient healing systems. It is one of the first things traditional Chinese doctors check into when you are examined. Western allopathic medicine is a relatively new system that has not yet taken this factor into account. Many new research studies have indicated that an acidic body is a disease-prone body. Otto Warberg, a two-time winner of the Nobel Prize for medicine, won one of his Nobel Prizes for proving that cancer is anaerobic. This means that cancer can only grow in acidic, oxygen-depleted bodies. Western medicine, however, has focused primarily on treating diseases after they manifest in the body. As modern medicine turns its primary attention to disease prevention, you will have a clearer picture of how important the acid/alkaline balance is for your radiant health and weight management.

Enough is known from prior experience and current studies for you to make your body's acid/alkaline balance a priority factor now. Controlling this balance is a relatively simple thing. Three main factors are involved: (1) your attitude, (2) food, and (3) nutrition. We have already talked about how our thoughts affect our body chemistry. Guess what? Certain thoughts make us more acidic and others make us more alkaline. The acidic thoughts fall under three main categories: "mad," "sad," and "scared." These three categories cover a wide range of specific emotions, from the extreme anger of hate to the extreme fearfulness of being panicked. On the other hand, alkaline thoughts fall under the category of "glad," which covers the entire range from total attunement to Divine Will Pleasure down to simple laughter at a funny joke. You may have heard of how laughter has influenced people's health and even contributed to the remission of cancer in some cases. When I did a website search of Amazon.com for books on "Laughter and Health," I received over 55,000 results. This is a lot to laugh about!

In previous chapters, we covered the discriminative process to go through in locating your dysfunctional beliefs and thoughts with regard to your weight. In this chapter, I am suggesting that you go one step further and discriminate to replace *all* thoughts that fall under the categories of "mad," "sad," and "scared." This will increase your alkalinity and increase your resistance to disease. Surely you can relate to the corrosive nature of these categories of negative thoughts, but you may not have known before that they actually have their own chemistry that is detrimental to your body. Of course, you can replace these acidic thoughts with the alkaline thoughts that fall under the category of "glad." So as the song goes, "Don't worry, be happy," and then you will be healthier, too.

Another factor affecting the acid/alkaline balance of your body is the food you eat. Many, and I do mean many, of the most commonly consumed foods today cause the body to become acidic. The foods having the most acidifying effect are foods you may consume the most, such as sodas, coffee, chips, artificial sweeteners, and corn syrup. Artificial sweeteners and corn syrup have slowly crept into about everything most people eat. These are some of the worst foods, but there are many more, including breads and most meat. Cigarettes and alcohol are very acidifying to the body as well.

Of course, you don't have to stop consuming these foods entirely. I still enjoy one cup of coffee a day, about two glasses of wine a week, and a small amount of chocolate every day. To restore your health, eat about 80 percent alkaline-forming foods and about 20 percent acid-forming foods until you reach the ideal pH goal. Once restored, maintain your health by eating about 60 percent alkaline-forming foods and 40 percent acid-forming foods.

The acid/alkaline pH scale runs from 0 (pure acid) to 14 (pure alkaline), with 7 as neutral. The goal is to have blood pH slightly alkaline, between 7.35 and 7.45, and all your other bodily fluids' pH between 6.50 and 7.45. You can test the pH of your body fluids with your saliva on litmus paper, usually obtained from the drug or healthfood store. Restoring the optimum balance will significantly contribute to a disease-resistant body. I have included a list of foods, and their acid/alkaline effect on your body, at the end of this book. (In the lists, you will see citrus fruit listed as "alkaline-forming." This is because stomach acid neutralizes the citric acid, leaving alkaline ash as the end result.)

Supplements also play a large role in achieving the correct acid/alkaline balance. I don't plan to go into depth here on supplements because there are plenty of places to get great information. I just want to mention briefly one factor—calcium. Calcium is one of the main controllers of the acid/alkaline balance for your body. Your body manufactures mono-ortho-calcium phosphate from calcium in the food and nutrients you consume. This compound acts as a crucial component of your body's pH buffering system. During the bonding process, when the compound is formed, alkaline salts of sodium and potassium also form. This calcium compound, along with the alkaline salts, maintains the body's proper alkalinity. Current biological research now links a large number of prevalent diseases to calcium deficiency. I believe that in the future, science will discover that this is due to the devastating corrosive effect of being overly acidic. There are several important factors that come into play to enable your body to absorb calcium. I recommend you do some nutritional research for yourself. It will be well-worth your time.

There is also evidence to suggest that the body disposes of excess acidic waste from the blood stream by storing it away in fatty tissue, so being overweight seems to be another side-effect of being too acidic.

An older gentleman I was sitting next to in a sauna said to me once, "If I had known I was going to live this long, I would have taken better care of myself." Do what it takes now so that you don't suffer illness or need to work hard in the future to correct what could have been prevented. Two sayings come to mind: "An ounce of prevention is worth a pound of cure," and "In addition to the years in your life, you also want life in your years."

If you want to create a disease free, radiantly healthy body, and achieve your ideal weight, then put time and attention on your acid/alkaline balance as part of your Intentional Weight Management. This is a powerful, empowering, and preventative step, which you can take for your radiant health.

Chapter 12

Exercise

There is such a wide range of benefits from regular exercise that the question should not be, "Do I exercise?" but, "How often do I exercise and how hard do I exercise as part of my Intentional Weight Management?" First let's look at the generally accepted benefits you receive from regular exercise, then at how often and how hard to work at it.

Many studies and books are available listing the benefits of exercise to your physical and mental well-being. The generally accepted benefits of regular exercise are: (1) reduced risk of premature death, (2) lower risk of heart disease, (3) less chance of high blood pressure, (4) reduced risk of colon cancer, breast cancer, and diabetes, (5) reduced or maintained body weight or body fat, (6) building and maintaining healthy muscles, bones, and joints, (7) reduced depression and anxiety, (8) improved psychological well-being, and (9) enhanced work, recreation, and sport performance. These are just a few, and I am sure there are many more.

An obvious benefit is that if we burn more calories than we take in, we will process weight off our bodies and get rid of it, but we don't want to take this to extremes because we could end up negatively impacting our radiant health. How can we safely determine how often and how hard we should work out? Briefly mentioned in "The Final Chapter," your blood type determines your own body type, which may guide you to the proper exercise. There are other systems out there that can also help you determine the best exercise suited for you and the frequency and force most beneficial for your body type, too. I would suggest that you at least examine the blood-typing system.

On the other hand, there is a previously discussed resource available for you to make this clear determination yourself: It is your heart! By getting in tune with the beat and pressure of your heart and tuning in to your total body, you will simply know! This process will reveal to you what type of exercise, how often to exercise and with what force to exercise for your radiant health and ideal weight. It's that simple.

I have noticed that many people over-exercise. I recommend staying in harmony and balance with the intelligence of your heart so you don't hurt yourself.

Exercise will help you process weight off your body and get rid of it. But getting overly attached to the concept of burning calories through exercise can be problematic. Conscious Awareness, used in the ways we have discussed, is the most powerful resource you have for creating a healthy body and achieving your ideal weight. It always comes down to mind over matter, so please honor your conscious awareness first. The power of that far exceeds any amount of exercise you could ever possibly do for creating your ideal body.

CNN.com posted an article entitled, "Studies: Walking Might Keep Mind Sharp." This article was a summary of several studies showing that regular, moderate walking helps prevent mental decline and Alzheimer's disease. The point is, you don't have to go to extremes. Find the right exercise for your body type. Determine how often and how hard you are going to do it. Then, make that exercise part of your Intentional Weight Management. This will contribute to the long-term success and overall quality of your journey.

The other resource is your Guardian Archangel who, when asked, is quite able to guide you. This guidance can come through direct realization or through books and people you meet who have information on exercise. Mysterious and magical are the ways of Divine Intervention, so ASK and then "stay alert." Answers will always show up in some way.

Chapter 13

Observed But Not "Proven"

Some things are observed to be true but no one has taken the time and effort to scientifically "prove" them to be true. In fact, we take many things for granted as true without ever seeing supporting scientific proof.

This happens to be the case with the next three things I am going to share with you. Time and time again, they have all been observed to be effective. I have put them all to the test of time through my own weight management work and can say without a shadow of doubt that they all work. These techniques have also been used by other people practicing in the healing arts and observed to be true with their clients.

The first of these techniques was discovered initially by observing the effects on injured people. Another of these techniques has been observed by Pavlov in his experiments with dogs, some of my favorite friends. Finally, the water crystal photography work by Masaru Emoto has gone a long way in adding scientific understanding as to how the third technique works.

The first technique is what I like to call, "Chewing your way through weight management." It has been observed that if you chew your food predominantly on the right side of your mouth, then you will process weight *on* to your body. If you chew your food predominantly on the left side of your mouth, then you will process weight *off* your body. It's that simple. I cannot explain how or why this works. I can, however, tell you it's worked for many people who have systematically employed this technique.

It has delighted me and surprised others when they observed the way they chew their food. In a significant number of cases, the overweight people chewed predominantly on the right and the underweight chewed predominantly on the left. I suggest that you first bring to your conscious awareness the way you are chewing your food now. By observing your natural tendency, you may be completely surprised to find this to be true in your case. Of course, if you inhale your food then you may not be able to prove this for yourself through immediate observation.

In any case, this is such a simple technique to use that it makes sense to personally put it to the test. Chew on the RIGHT TO INCREASE weight. Chew on the LEFT TO DECREASE weight. That's all there is to it. So, like I said, "Chew your way through weight management."

I call the second technique "Following the scent of weight management." This very simple technique involves using your nose. Basically, the secret is getting a good whiff of what you're eating. By this I mean smelling your food. Before you start eating, it is very important to smell your food. During the time you are eating, stop every once in a while and smell your food. Even when you are chewing your food, you can inhale through your nose with the intention of smelling the food you are chewing as well as what's on your plate.

There are many reasons for doing this. First, it's very pleasing to smell your food. You will be much more satisfied from smelling in addition to chewing and swallowing it. Second, you will digest your food better, therefore absorbing more of its nutritional value. These effects will result in being more satisfied and having fewer food cravings.

I used to always finish what was on my plate. I also almost always took a second portion before I would be finished at any meal. Once I started smelling my food, not only did I stop taking second portions, sometimes I even left food on my plate from the first portion. This was very surprising to me and contributes significantly to my personal weight management.

There are some scientific bases for understanding why this may work. During the time when Pavlov was experimenting with dogs, he did one experiment that may give some clues. He cut dogs' stomachs open and placed food directly into them to observe what happened to the food. (These dogs where alive and remained alive for the experimentation.) He observed that the food sat there for a long time while the stomach basically did little with it. Next, he did the same thing except this time he placed some of the food in front of the dogs' noses and let the dogs begin to smell the food but not eat it. He observed that the dogs' stomachs immediately started the process of digesting the food that had been placed directly in their stomachs.

This shows a direct correlation between digesting food and smelling it ... at least in dogs. I have found it to be true for humans as well that the aroma of food will affect your appetite and help increase the absorption of the nutrition in your food. So, as simple as it is, why not "Follow the scent of weight management?"

I call the last technique "My personal pharmacy." It has been observed that the conscious awareness we bring to anything will alter that thing. I have previously mentioned this "uncertainty principle" by which the act of looking at an electron changes its position and/or speed. This same principle of altering things with the power of our thoughts can be applied to food.

Imagine all the possibilities that this opens up. We can enhance the quality of the food we eat in many ways. We can direct the nutrition from the food to a specific area of the body to accelerate healing. We can enhance our meal to support our weight management. With conscious awareness and specific intention, we can turn our food into healing substances for a radiant healthy ideal body.

This principle regarding the food we eat has been used and observed by wise individuals for thousands of years. Within the last several decades, the research of Masaru Emoto has given us a clear picture of this in water. Mr. Emoto has spent the majority of his life researching water and the effects of conscious awareness and specific intention upon it.

In his book, *The Hidden Messages in Water*, Masaru demonstrates how thoughts, feeling, words and music structure water in very specific ways. Through exposing water to different words such as "gratitude," "love," "wisdom," "fool," "hate" and "Satan," he has demonstrated how they effect the structure of water. He has demonstrated this by freezing the exposed water and taking pictures of the different crystal structures that form. The photographs of these structures are strikingly different, I would say enlightening. (You can see many of the photos on his website at: www.masaru-emoto.net/english/entop.html)

Our bodies and the food we put into them are about 70 percent water. So we can simply change the structure of the food we put into our bodies and turn them into specific substances to help heal and reshape our bodies. This is done by the thoughts we fill our food with before we eat it. Before eating, I take time to embrace my food with thoughts of gratitude and love. I then embrace the meal with thoughts and feelings of "radiant health" and "ideal weight." If I have any specific area of my body where I feel pain, I also have thoughts of healing nutrition from the meal going specifically into that area of my body.

This is the ultimate pharmacopoeia and it does not cost you an extra dime. It may be hard to believe but it has been observed to work wonderfully. You too can have your own "personal pharmacy" every time you sit down to a meal.

By the way, if you think a food is fattening, it will be. So make a conscious choice about not only what you put into your body but also what you're thinking about as you put it in. Your thoughts and intention will make a huge or small difference.

Chapter 14

Diets Don't Work

Diets don't work for long-term health or Intentional Weight Management. They don't work because we are creatures of habit. Unless you want to create a habit of dieting the rest of your life, you can forget all about it. I am sure you know some people who diet their whole lives. But come on, "are they having fun yet?" Most likely not. In fact, they are probably doing that weight-bouncing thing, going up and down like a yo-yo. They never really get healthy or achieve their ideal weight for any sustained period.

If you are going to succeed at anything, you must be joyful while doing it. You must be in love with what you are doing to really enjoy it and sustain it.

Love is your power, your creative driving force. I can say without a doubt that I love making and eating chocolate truffles. Do you know anyone who can say that about dieting? If they can, more power to them, but I have not met one yet.

The point is, first you must make a habit of the things you have already discovered in this book. "As above, so below." Make a habit of handling it within the super-substance of mind first, and the rest will follow. Make a habit of deepening and expanding your conscious awareness through meditation. Make a habit of discriminating about your total language. Make a habit out of focusing your conscious awareness in the positive ways already discussed about acid/alkaline thinking. These habits will serve you very well in achieving a "sound mind and body beaming with brightness," and manifesting your ideal weight. If you make these habits, as I have, then you will easily have the long-term health and ideal weight you desire. These habits will assist you in all areas of your life; you can count on it.

At the same time, you can definitely make a habit of certain types of eating styles that will promote your health from the outside, too. "Burning the candle at both ends" does produce quicker, long-lasting results. I spent many years fine-tuning the eating habits I have today. These eating habits promote my overall health and ideal weight, and have contributed significantly to my long-term success.

We have already discussed adopting a supplement program, the vital energetic component of food, how important it is to keep your body alkaline, and how exercise can help. These are all external things that will help you tremendously in your long-term success.

"The Final Chapter" discusses the cutting edge of eating technology—a unique eating technology founded on rock solid scientific investigation. It is not a fad and it surely is not a way of dieting. It is a way of eating scientifically, based on simple principles that will promote your long-term health and ideal weight. Once you understand these principles, then it is easy to apply this unique technology specifically to your body type.

One of my hobbies is gourmet cooking, and I love cooking all kinds of food. I especially love to bake anything chocolate. Besides cooking and baking, I love to make chocolate candy. Chocolate truffles are a specialty of mine. Today I had two chocolate truffles with my lunch that I made with 50-year-old plum brandy from Czechoslovakia, so you must realize I don't diet! But I do have a precise style of eating that is habitual. This allows me to enjoy eating while maintaining a healthy body and my ideal weight. This is one of the gifts in this book, "Joyful Eating."

Chapter 15

Adding Weight, Also

This chapter is for people who need to "process weight onto their body and keep it." If that is not you, please skip to the next chapter. If you are one of those rare individuals who need to process weight onto your body and keep it, Intentional Weight Management is for you, too. All the resources in this book are for the purpose of creating radiant health and achieving your ideal weight. This means that if you apply them, with some minor adjustments, every resource presented will help you process weight onto your body and keep it. Let me show you what I mean.

In Chapter 7, we saw how language shapes your attention and manifests your reality. If you are under-

weight, for your radiant health and ideal weight, you could use these phrases:
- "Processing weight onto my body and keeping it."
- "Processed weight onto my body and kept it."

These phrases will help you with your long-term weight management. Your heart and Guardian Archangel, discussed in Chapter 9 may guide you to an even better phrase for you. From these examples, you get the idea of the direction you need to go in.

The Radiant Health Process in Chapter 6 is going to help you in ways you cannot imagine at this time. A "sound mind and body beaming with brightness" is not a gaunt, thin, out-of-proportion body. It is a body of ideal weight, whatever that weight might be, for your body type.

Chapter 8, which contains the sutra meditation technique for regulating appetite, will help you, too. Simply substitute the phrase "Strength of an Elephant" for "Trachea". This will spontaneously increase your appetite and add body mass. Once you practice it as recommended, you will find yourself eating just the right amount of food for your radiant health and ideal weight. This technique is very powerful for those with problematic appetites that are too small for their bodies.

Attention to your body's acidic/alkaline balance will definitely help your weight. "The Final Chapter" will help you process weight onto your body and keep it by providing you with some additional resources on the most powerful eating technology available for your body type. It will allow you to select the right foods for you and the exercise best suited for you. This certainly can result in "processing weight onto your body and keeping it" and help you with your radiant health.

Meditation, discrimination, and the use of the "super-substance of mind" will allow you to achieve harmony and balance. This will be reflected in the way your body presents itself. Again, *ask* your Guardian Archangel for help and guidance. It will definitely assist you. Its entire purpose to help you with every aspect of your life, and that includes processing weight onto your body and keeping it if that is what is needed.

The information in Chapter 13 is especially important. There is no reason why you can't: "Chew your way through weight management," "Follow the scent of weight management," and use "Your personal pharmacy." You will greatly benefit from the effects of these three simple techniques.

The bottom line for you is the same as anyone who wants to process weight off his or her body and get rid of it. Make a habit of using all the resources of the Intentional Weight Management program. When you do, you will create radiant health and achieve your ideal weight. Remember, your radiant health and ideal weight do not depend solely upon the food you eat. The vital energy force you allow into your bodies contributes immensely.

Chapter 16

The Final Chapter

By making all the previously mentioned resources into habits, I achieved great success. My body was much healthier and my weight normalized. I had lots more energy, looked and felt much better, and was having lots of fun. I felt much freer to enjoy eating, and socializing became enjoyable. My life was working on many levels and I was "glad" most of the time.

At the same time, my conscious awareness was always seeking new information that would help me refine my eating habits. I was always interested in improving upon what I knew and empowering myself even more. Fortunately, I had built relationships with master healers and continually communicated with them, incorporating their recommendations into my life style. One day, a doctor friend of mine suggested to me how I could use the latest and greatest eating technology to improve my health further and gain even more energy.

Knowing that diets don't work, and having a desire to improve on my eating habits, I was enthusiastic to hear that and ready to go to the next level. Please realize the contents of this book so far offer a complete system that will get you to a self-sufficient place with your radiant health and ideal weight. But this final chapter will move you to the ultimate level in creating radiant health and in achieving your ideal weight.

The technology turned out to be the ultimate fine-tuning, the combination of two eating technologies into one system. This was a new and unique approach to eating that had not been previously available to the general pubic before the publication of two books. Creating a new style of eating turned out to be simpler than I had imagined. It also gave me the freedom to enjoy eating some of my favorite foods whenever I wanted. After about a month of eating this way, I noticed a definite improvement in my radiant health and my ideal body weight.

The two books that I read are, *Mastering the Zone*, by Barry Sears, Ph.D., and *Eat Right 4 Your Type*, by Dr. Peter J. D'Adamo. Neither of these books are "diet" or "fad" books. They both address a style of eating that you can easily maintain for your whole life.

They are about eating in a way that keeps you at the peak of your performance and feeling good physically and mentally. Finally, they are time-tested eating styles that do not limit your ability to enjoy the pleasures of food.

If you have never read Dr. Sears's book, you may have some misconceptions about it. His concept of "Zone" eating is not high protein and low or no carbohydrate eating. It is naturally balanced eating! For a long time, I ate too much protein and did not create a radiantly healthy body or achieve my ideal weight. High protein meals made me mentally and physically sluggish, constipated, and unable to reach my ideal weight.

"Zone" eating is based on scientific research of your body's hormonal response to food. This was discovered in Nobel Prize research into how aspirin works in your body to control pain. It also happens to be how humans ate for thousands of years before the advent of our modern food production and processing. Once understood, this "age old eating" is an easy to apply eating style that anyone can make into a habit. It is a way of combining specific proportions of carbohydrate, protein, and fat at every meal to obtain a beneficial hormonal response, and it is something you can do for the rest of your life.

One valuable piece of information gleaned from reading *Mastering the Zone* has been how fat actually controls appetite. Have you ever noticed how people who are on fat-free diets are always hungry and have strong cravings? When you read, *Mastering the Zone*, you will understand the reason for this. I have made fat my friend and have lots of fun using dark chocolate, which is low in sugar and high in fat, to help control my appetite.

The information in *Eat Right 4 Your Type* is based on two generations of scientific research. It is an easy-to-understand book based on the fact that not everybody should eat the same things or do the same exercises. The beauty of it is, all you need to know is your blood type. Based on that information, you can follow the recommended foods and exercises for your type. I have had remarkable results following these recommendations for my blood type.

Some foods I used to eat did not agree with me. I did not know why after some meals, I would feel sick or run down. At times, I would have heartburn or feel bloated. Other times, I would get very sleepy or agitated. When I started making a habit of eating the foods appropriate for my blood type, these symptoms simply did not occur anymore. This knowledge has been of great benefit to me and it will be for you also.

The beauty of these two books is that they both have tables to follow that make applying the information very clear. They are well-written, well-organized, and very user-friendly, making the combining of the information a thoroughly enjoyable task.

I recommend you use the proper proportions carbohydrates, protein, and fat from *Mastering the Zone* eating technology with the food appropriate to your blood type as prescribed in *Eat Right 4 Your Type* eating technology. Once you understand these principles, it is just a matter of referring to the tables within both books. Soon you won't even have to look at the tables; knowing what and how to combine the foods you eat at each meal will have become a habit. You will also know the ideal amount of food to eat at each meal.

By making a habit of all the previous resources called, Intentional Weight Management, I was led in this direction. It is the last step and ultimate fine-tuning that has helped me to create radiant health and achieve my ideal weight. The powerful uniqueness created by the synergy of these two systems builds a habit of eating more beneficially than either of them does separately. I perform better, feel better, and easily sustain radiant health and my ideal weight. I have demonstrated long-term success for years now.

The whole purpose of this chapter is to inspire you. By using these systems together, I got to my complete, joyful destination regarding my radiant health and ideal weight. Once you have read *Mastering the Zone* and *Eat Right 4 Your Type*, combine the information and apply it towards your habitual style of eating. It will give you greater freedom to enjoy eating and help to sustain your long-term results. It is a powerful supplement to the resources contained within this book.

Epilogue

Achieving Your Goals

Congratulations! You have successfully come to the conclusion of this book. You have a wide range of resources that constitute the system of Intentional Weight Management. Separately, each of these resources will help you improve your radiant health and achieve your ideal weight. Together the power of these resources is exponential in getting you there with "God's Speed" and sustaining those results over the course of your life. You will find that once you habitually use these resources, the amount of effort you put into your Intentional Weight Management will be far less than you have exerted in the past with other methods. At the same time, the long-term results will be far greater.

If you don't use these resources or you use them sporadically, you will not get the swift, long-term results others and myself have obtained. I have covered a wide range of resources, from meditation to exercise. Making a habit of all of these requires focus and follow-through. In the beginning, it takes more time and attention; but once these resources become familiar habits, then you will be surprised as to how effortlessly you use them.

I found it takes "The Four Wheels," as I call them, to move through this process and make using these resources a familiar habit for achieving your goals. These four wheels are: Commitment, Devotion, Faith, and Courage:

- Without your *commitment* to your goal and to utilizing these resources, nothing can be accomplished. Commitment produces the focusing power behind your energy of intention. As your first step, you must make a commitment, if you expect results.

- *Devotion* keeps you in love with the idea and the picture of a "sound mind and body beaming with brightness" and continually brings you back to your goal and resources time and time again, no matter what distractions arise.

- *Faith* keeps you relaxed and at peace, adding flexibility to the flow of your energies while using your resources to achieve your goal. This flexibility allows your conscious awareness spontaneously to take in all available information and process it for use in the manifestation of your intentions.

- Courage keeps you pursuing your goals even in the face of obstacles. It gives you the power to overcome these obstacles and realize the opportunities hidden within them.

"The Four Wheels" will keep you moving forward on your life's journey, efficiently and effectively. It has been my experience that whenever my life seemed to break down, I stopped moving forward because at least one of "The Four Wheels" (commitment, devotion, faith, courage) was weak, and I was like a car with a flat tire. Then to get my life back on the road, I had to determine which one or ones were weak and do the work necessary to re-energize and strengthen them. Once that was accomplished, I got back on the road and moved forward rather quickly.

My final recommendations are:

- Make a commitment to your radiant health, ideal weight and a habit of using the resources available to you.
- Fall in love with the idea and the images of your radiant health, ideal weight and the use of your resources. A "sound mind and body beaming with brightness" is something you can be devoted to.
- Have faith in the resources presented in this book, especially your Guardian Archangel,

and your ability to use them to achieve your radiant health and ideal weight.

- Meet whatever obstacles present themselves with courage. Have the intention to realize the meaning behind the obstacles and utilize them as opportunities.

Please remember that many of the resources in this book can be used to achieve any goal in your life's journey. Your heart, along with your Guardian Archangel, will guide you in developing the language you need to shape the quality of your attention towards accomplishing any end. Numerous resources presented in this book, when made familiar habits, will improve the quality of all areas of your life simultaneously. Putting "The Four Wheels" into action on the road of your life's journey will gracefully carry you to your joyful destination. "When your understanding changes so does your direction." Now you are ready to head off in a new direction with a little help from your angelic friends.

Contract With Myself for Achieving Radiant Health & My Ideal Weight

I, _____, commit to my radiant health, ideal weight, and habit of using the resources available to me through Intentional Weight Management as well as any other resources brought to me by Divine Intervention.

I devote myself to the idea and images of my radiant health, ideal weight, and the use of all available resources. I have fallen in love with my "sound mind and body beaming with brightness" and the habits that successfully achieve and maintain that goal.

I have faith in the resources presented in this book, especially my Guardian Archangel. I also have faith in my own ability to use these resources to achieve and maintain my radiant health and ideal weight. I trust in the Total Wisdom, Total Power, and Total Love of God to assist me in achieving my goals.

I will meet with courage whatever obstacles that present themselves, and have the intention to realize the meaning behind those obstacles. I will courageously use any obstacles as opportunities to achieve and maintain my radiant health and ideal weight.

Upon signing this contract today, I bring the full force of my commitment, devotion, faith, and courage forward to achieve and maintain a "sound mind and body beaming with brightness."

Signed: _____ Date: _____

Appendix: Acid/Alkaline Foods

Very Alkaline-Forming:
Emotional Category: "glad"

Cantaloupe, Cayenne (Capsicum), Dried dates & figs, Kelp, Karengo, Kudzu root, Lemons, Limes, Mango, Melons, Papaya, Parsley, Seedless grapes (sweet), Watercress, Seaweeds, Asparagus, Endive, Kiwifruit, Fruit juices, Grapes (sweet), Passion fruit, Pears (sweet), Pineapple, Raisins, Umeboshi plum, Vegetable juices, Watermelon.

Moderately Alkaline-forming:

Apples (sweet), Apples (sour), Apricots, Alfalfa sprouts, Arrowroot flour, Avocados, Bamboo shoots, Bananas (ripe), Beans (fresh green), Beets, Bell Pepper, Berries, Broccoli, Cabbage, Carob, Carrots, Celery, Currants, Daikon, Dates & figs (fresh), Garlic, Ginger (fresh), Gooseberry, Grapes (less sweet), Grapes (sour), Grapefruit, Guavas, Herbs (leafy green), Kale, Kohlrabi, Lettuce (leafy green), Lettuce (pale green), Nectarine, Peaches (sweet), Oranges, Parsnip, Peaches (less sweet), Pears (less sweet), Peas fresh sweet), Peas (less sweet), Persimmon, Potatoes & skin, Pumpkin (sweet), Pumpkin (less sweet), Raspberry, Sea salt, Spinach, Strawberry, Squash, Sweet corn (fresh), Tamari, Turnip, Vinegar (apple cider).

Slightly Alkaline-forming:

Almonds, Amaranth, Artichokes (Jerusalem), Artichoke (globe), Barley-Malt (sweetener-Bronner), Brown Rice Syrup, Brussel Sprouts, Cherries, Chestnuts (dry roasted), Coconut (fresh), Cucumbers, Eggplant, Egg yolks (soft cooked), Essene bread, Goat's milk and whey (raw), Honey (raw), Horseradish, Leeks, Mayonnaise (home made), Millet, Miso, Mushrooms, Okra, Olive oil, Olives ripe, Onions, Pickles, (home made), Quinoa, Radish, Rhubarb, Sesame seeds (whole), Soy beans (dry), Soy cheese, Soy milk, Spices, Sprouted grains, Taro, Tempeh, Tofu, Tomatoes (sweet), Tomatoes (less sweet), Vinegar (sweet brown rice), Water Chestnut, Yeast (nutritional flakes).

Neutral-forming:

Butter (fresh unsalted), Cream (fresh & raw), Milk (raw cow's), Oils (except olive), Whey, Yogurt (plain).

Slightly Acid-forming:

Barley malt syrup, Barley, Bran, Cashews, Cereals (unrefined with honey-fruit-maple syrup), Cornmeal, Cranberries, Fructose, Honey (pasteurized), Lentils, Macadamias, Maple syrup (unprocessed), Milk (homogenized) and most processed dairy products, Molasses (unsulphered organic), Nutmeg, Mustard, Pistachios, Popcorn & butter (plain), Rice or wheat crackers (unrefined), Rye (grain), Rye bread (organic sprouted), Seeds (pumpkin & sunflower), Walnuts, Blueberries, Brazil nuts, Butter (salted), Cheeses (mild & crumbly),

Crackers (unrefined rye), Dried beans (mung, adzuki, pinto, kidney, garbanzo), Dry coconut, Egg whites, Goats milk (homogenized), Olives (pickled), Pecans, Plums, Prunes, Spelt.

Moderately Acid-forming:

Bananas (green), Breads (refined) of corn, oats, rice & rye, Buckwheat, Cereals (refined), Corn flakes, Cheeses (sharp), Cigarette tobacco (roll your own), Corn & Rice breads, Cream of Wheat (unrefined), Egg whole (cooked hard), Fish, Fruit juices with sugar, Ketchup, Maple syrup (processed), Mayonnaise, Molasses (sulphured), Oats, Pasta (whole grain), Pastry (whole grain), Peanuts, Pickles (commercial), Potatoes (with no skins), Popcorn (with salt & butter), Rice (basmati), Rice (brown), Shellfish, Wheat germ, Soy sauce (commercial), Tapioca, Wheat bread (sprouted organic), Whole Wheat foods, Wine, Yogurt (sweetened).

Extremely Acid-forming:

Emotional Categories: "mad, sad, scared"

Artificial sweeteners, Beef, Carbonated soft drinks & fizzy drinks, Cigarettes (tailor made), Drugs, Flour (white or wheat), Goat, Lamb, Pastries & Cakes from white flour, Pork, Sugar (white) Beer, Brown sugar, Chicken, Deer, Chocolate, Coffee, Custard with white sugar, Jams, Jellies, Liquor, Pasta (white), Rabbit, Semolina, Table salt refined & iodized, Tea (black), Turkey, White bread, White rice, White vinegar (processed).

About the Author

Mahesh Subrahmanyam's life direction is very different today than it was 32 years ago. His life has turned out totally different than anyone back then predicted. When asked, Mahesh attributes it to an event he labels his "Wake Up Call" and the choices he has made ever since.

It was Memorial Day weekend in 1973 when the call came. That call was delivered when, driving a motorcycle, he hit a telephone pole straight on at 60 miles per hour. He died and, on "the other side," he was taken on a journey that revealed the nature of our connectedness among all things and many other mysteries. At the end of this process, he was given a choice to move on or return to the earth to fulfill his original contract. The realization from that experience changed the course of his life forever.

Obviously he chose to return but, to return, he had to change course and follow the destiny of his original contract. He says, "At the time of the call, I was way off course and feel deeply fortunate to have been given a second chance. It's funny that when I was called, God actually used a 'telephone-pole.' I guess long-distance is the next best thing to being there."

Mahesh believes that our life experience has everything to do with our motivation and intentionality. "How we put our conscious awareness to use is of the utmost importance. Inherent in our connectivity is a far-reaching influence that affects everything in creation, seen and unseen. It is our destiny as children of God to support and uplift all of God's Creation. God has given us the Divine Tool of Consciousness itself to be used for this purpose."

He is dedicated to developing conscious awareness to its fullest extent and using whatever gifts that brings to assist in our global evolution. This has been his path for the last 32 years, a path he finds not always easy, but simple and deeply rewarding. From this fertile ground, the current book *Intention Weight Management* has grown.

Printed in the United States
27548LVS00001BB/157-246